S.O.S.
SURVIVAL OR STRATEGY – HOW TO COACH YOUR DAMN SELF

By Clifton John Roy Jr.

COPYRIGHT PAGE

Published by:

PEN Business Solutions

Lafayette, Louisiana

www.penbusinesssolutions.com

info@penbusinesssolutions.com

Title: S.O.S.: Survival or Strategy – How To Coach Your Damn Self

Author: Clifton John Roy Jr.

Cover Design: Clifton John Roy Jr.

Interior Layout: Self-Designed

ISBN: 979-8-9993239-0-3

First Edition: 2025

For permissions, licensing, bulk orders, or speaking engagements, contact:

info@penbusinesssolutions.com

Printed in the United States of America.

LEGAL DISCLAIMER

The content of this book is intended to provide general guidance and empowerment based on the author's experiences and coaching frameworks. It is not intended as a substitute for medical, legal, financial, or psychological advice. Always seek professional help from qualified practitioners before making significant decisions affecting your health, finances, or well-being. The author and publisher disclaim any liability for any losses or damages incurred in connection with the use of this content.

COACHING STATEMENT

This book was created to empower individuals to take full ownership of their personal growth journey. While it draws from coaching principles, it is not intended to replace one-on-one coaching or therapy. S.O.S. is a self-guided system to help you reflect, plan, and take action—but your growth is yours to own. If deeper personal transformation is needed, seek a certified coach, therapist, or support professional. This book is here to help you get real, not stay stuck.

DEDICATION

This book is dedicated to every soul who's ever been stuck between who they are and who they were born to be.

To the ones who learned how to survive—but never got the blueprint to build.

To the ones who had to coach themselves through silent battles.

To the cycle breakers. The inner healers. The dreamers with bruises.

To the version of me that didn't quit—and the version of you that refuses to go back.

You are not broken. You are becoming.

And this book is for you.

TABLE OF CONTENTS

INTRODUCTION

I didn't write this book because I had everything figured out.

I wrote this book because I didn't.

Because like you, I've faced days when I didn't recognize myself in the mirror. Nights when I questioned why I was still here. And seasons when I gave the best advice to others—but forgot how to apply it to myself.

See, I was raised by a man who wanted me to be better than him—not like him. My father, with all his faults and all his love, planted that seed early: "Go further than I did. Stand taller." I carried that mission with me through trauma I never expected—like being molested by my aunt and made to believe it was normal. That kind of betrayal rewires something in you. It doesn't just hurt—it shapes you.

At 17, I made a decision that would change everything. I joined the U.S. Army. My parents had to sign off because I wasn't even legally old enough to go alone. But I went—because I didn't want my dreams of going to college to become a financial burden on my family. I wanted to protect my siblings from that pressure. So I chose service.

I traveled the world, grew up fast, learned discipline, leadership, and silence. I returned to Louisiana in 2002 after leaving in 1993—something I swore I'd never do. But life has a funny way of circling you back to the places you tried to outrun. And for years, I struggled to find my footing. I broke—not just emotionally, but mentally, spiritually, and eventually, physically.

> " Then came the brain surgery. The reset I didn't ask for... "

Then came the brain surgery. The reset I didn't ask for—but the one that made everything stop.

It was during the long, slow climb after surgery—2 and a half years into recovery—that something clicked: all the insight I had given to others... all the tools I had used to help people heal, lead, grow, and transform... I needed them too. And for the first time in my life, I turned all that love and leadership inward.

I became my own coach.

And that's why Coach Your Damn Self exists—not just for the entrepreneur, the single mom, the person of faith, or the everyday survivor—but for the version of me who was tired of suffering in silence. For the version of you who's ready to stop pretending, stop settling, and start doing the work that will finally set you free.

WHAT YOU'LL LEARN IN THIS BOOK

This book is your guide. It doesn't promise perfection, but it will walk you through the powerful truth that everything you need to grow already exists inside of you.

We'll start by understanding the six parts of your whole self—your **P.I.E.S.E.S.**:

- ➢ **Physical** – your health, energy, and body
- ➢ **Intellectual** – your learning, thinking, and beliefs
- ➢ **Emotional** – your ability to feel and process
- ➢ **Social** – your relationships and support systems
- ➢ **Economical** – your finances and resources
- ➢ **Spiritual** – your connection to purpose and higher calling

> **...know exactly what's helping you grow and what's holding you back.**

You'll then complete a **S.W.O.T. analysis**—breaking down your Strengths, Weaknesses, Opportunities, and Threats based on your **P.I.E.S.E.S**.—so you know exactly what's helping you grow and what's holding you back.

We'll walk through the emotional toll of change using the **D.A.B.D.A.** grief model—Denial, Anger, Bargaining, Depression, and Acceptance—because becoming new means saying goodbye to parts of your old self.

From there, we'll set real goals using the **S.M.A.R.T.** framework—Specific, Measurable, Attainable, Realistic, and Timely—so you're not just dreaming... you're moving.

> **Your future is being written by your thoughts.**

You'll also explore the why behind your choices by unpacking the **T.A.H.C.D.** process— *Thought → Action → Habit → Character → Destiny.* Your future is being written by your thoughts. Change your thinking, and you can rewrite your destiny.

Finally, you'll learn how to do the work with the **I.D.E.A.L.S.O.L.V.E.** system:

- ➢ Identify the real issue
- ➢ Define your goals
- ➢ Explore solutions
- ➢ Assess what's needed
- ➢ Layout your plan

- ➤ Start taking action
- ➤ Observe the process
- ➤ Look for gaps
- ➤ Verify your results
- ➤ Evolve into the highest version of you

Let's Be Real

This book is raw. It's honest. It's not sugarcoated. I'm not here to impress you—I'm here to help you.

You'll feel challenged. You'll feel exposed. But you'll also feel seen. Heard. Empowered.

And most importantly, you'll be reminded that you've always had what it takes. You just needed someone to speak your language, walk beside you, and call out the greatness in you.

That's what I'm here for.

Let's coach your damn self—and change your life for good.

CHAPTER 1: PHYSICAL – THE FOUNDATION OF YOU

Before we can talk about purpose, profit, peace, or progress—we've got to talk about the body.

Your body is the first coach you'll ever have. It speaks before your mind forms words. It tells you when to rest, when to move, when something's off, and when something's on fire inside of you. But too many of us learn to ignore those signals—until our body screams.

When I talk about the Physical dimension of who you are, I'm not just talking about weight or appearance. I'm talking about three layers of your physical self:

- ➢ **External** – What people can see
- ➢ **Internal** – What only you and your body know
- ➢ **Perception** – What you believe about your physical health

Let's break that down.

THE EXTERNAL: WHAT THE WORLD SEES

This is the layer most people focus on first. How you look. How you walk into a room. Your energy, posture, grooming, even the clothes you wear.

> **People don't see your spirit first—they see your body.**

And while that's not everything, it does matter. **People don't see your spirit first—they see your body.** They hear your voice. They feel your presence.

Ask yourself:

➢ Does the way I show up match the life I say I want?
➢ Do I look like I care about myself?

What is my body language saying about my confidence, boundaries, and self-worth?

You don't have to fit into society's mold of beauty or strength. But you do have to own the message your body is sending.

THE INTERNAL: WHAT'S REALLY GOING ON

You can look good and still feel like hell on the inside.

What's happening in your body that nobody sees? High blood pressure? Gut issues? Fatigue? Chronic pain? Many of us were raised in environments where we pushed through illness, ignored symptoms, or called it "just stress." But your body is always trying to tell you the truth— even if you've trained yourself not to listen.

Let me be transparent: I didn't take my internal health seriously until I had no choice. **Brain surgery was my wake-up call.** And in recovery, I realized just how much damage I had tolerated, avoided, and minimized. Don't wait for your body to shut down to start paying attention.

> **Brain surgery was my wake-up call.**

Reflect on:

> ➤ How often do I feel tired, sick, or "off"?

➤ Do I sleep well? Eat like I care about myself? Move with intention?

➤ Have I made peace with going to the doctor, or do I avoid checkups like the plague?

➤ Ignoring internal issues won't make them go away. It only postpones the confrontation—and raises the cost of recovery.

PERCEPTION: WHAT YOU THINK ABOUT YOUR BODY

Now let's get personal. Because you can eat kale, run five miles, and still hate what you see in the mirror. Or you can avoid the mirror altogether.

How you feel about your body affects **every decision you make**. It determines the clothes you wear, the relationships you tolerate, the way you show up for opportunities, and the limits you place on yourself.

Sometimes, your body isn't the problem. Your **perspective** is.

Ask yourself:

- ➢ Do I speak about my body with kindness or criticism?
- ➢ What beliefs about my body did I inherit from family, culture, trauma?
- ➢ Am I taking care of my body—or punishing it?

REAL TALK: THIS IS THE BASE OF THE PYRAMID

If you don't have the energy to get up, think clearly, or follow through—it's going to be hard to change your life. Period. The Physical dimension is the foundation for your P.I.E.S.E.S. because everything else stacks on top of it.

This chapter isn't here to shame you—it's here to wake you up. You don't need to look like a model or eat salads 24/7. But you do need to start treating your body like the first business you manage. You wouldn't run a company and never check your equipment, tools, or systems. Your body is your system. It is suppose to carry you to and into your purpose.

Let's Do the Work

Take some time to evaluate your physical self through these prompts:

- ➢ What is one thing I can do today to honor my body?
- ➢ What am I ignoring physically that needs my attention?
- ➢ How would I show up differently if I felt physically strong, rested, and energized?
- ➢ What small routines (water, sleep, movement) could I commit to right now?

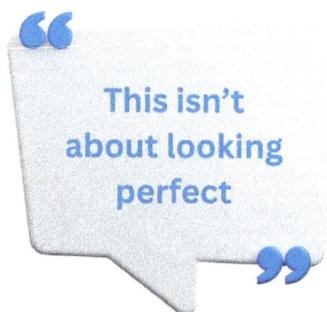

> **This isn't about looking perfect**

This isn't about looking perfect. It's about getting real with yourself and building a body that supports the vision you've been praying, planning, and pushing for.

Your next level doesn't need a new wardrobe—it needs a new commitment to your physical well-being.

Coach your body. Then let your body show the world how ready you are.

CHAPTER 2: INTELLECTUAL – THE POWER OF YOUR MIND

You've heard the phrase, **"Change your mind, change your life."** But let me be real with you—it's not just a catchy quote. It's a law.

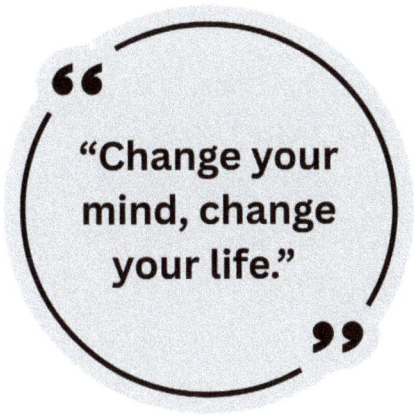

> **"Change your mind, change your life."**

Your mind is your steering wheel. And if your thoughts are out of alignment, don't be surprised if your life keeps swerving off course.

The Intellectual dimension of your life is all about how you think, learn, grow, and challenge yourself. It's your capacity to take in new information, question old beliefs, and make smart, strategic decisions that move you forward. It's the mental sharpness that fuels your creativity, your problem-solving, your ability to plan, and your resilience when life hits hard.

This chapter is about checking the condition of your mind—not just your memory or intelligence, but your willingness to grow intellectually even when it's uncomfortable.

WHAT DOES "INTELLECTUAL" REALLY MEAN?

It doesn't mean you have to be a genius, get straight A's, or love reading 300-page books (unless you want to). It means you're aware of what's happening between your ears—and you're intentional about what you do with it.

It's:

➢ What you feed your mind (media, conversation, books, ideas)
➢ How you process what happens to you
➢ Whether you let fear or facts lead your decisions
➢ Whether your thinking is building your future—or blocking it

THE MENTAL LOOPS YOU KEEP RUNNING

Most of us live on mental autopilot. We think what we've always thought. We react the way we've always reacted. We chase goals that aren't even ours anymore because we never stop to ask, "Why do I believe this?"

> **"But if you never filter what stays, you'll live your life based on assumptions, trauma, and someone else's truth"**

Your brain is always collecting information. But if you never filter what stays, you'll live your life based on assumptions, trauma, and someone else's truth.

Ask yourself:

- ➤ What thoughts do I repeat daily that don't serve me?
- ➤ Who taught me what I currently believe about success, failure, relationships, or money?

> ➢ Do I challenge my thoughts—or just follow them?

THE GROWTH (OR STAGNATION) YOU ALLOW

Some of us haven't upgraded our mindset since high school. We're still operating on survival logic. Still reacting based on what worked during the struggle, not what's needed for our next level. If you want your life to evolve, your thinking has to grow first.

And growth doesn't happen by accident. You have to seek it. Feed it. Protect it.

Start here:

> ➢ Are you reading things that sharpen you?
> ➢ Are you around people who stretch your thinking or shrink it?
> ➢ Do you give yourself time to think—or just react?

Intellectual growth means you stop being a sponge and start being a filter. Not every thought belongs. Not every belief is worth keeping. You have the right—and the responsibility—to upgrade.

MENTAL DISCIPLINE IS SELF-DEFENSE

A weak mind is a wide-open door for stress, fear, anxiety, and manipulation. But a strong, disciplined mind? That's armor.

When you build intellectual discipline, you become harder to shake, easier to focus, and quicker to recover from emotional storms. You don't just react to life—you respond with strategy.

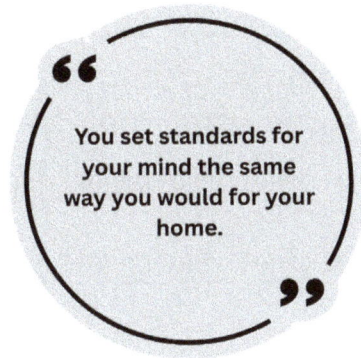

> " **You set standards for your mind the same way you would for your home.** "

That's how you coach your damn self. You don't let every thought run wild. **You set standards for your mind the same way you would for your home.**

REAL TALK: STOP LETTING OLD THOUGHTS WRITE YOUR NEW LIFE

Let me say this with love and fire: Some of y'all are praying for a new season with an old mindset. That won't work. You want new results? You need new thoughts. I have always said that you can't fix a problem with the same mind that created it.

And don't get it twisted—healing your thinking doesn't always feel good. It means questioning the things you were taught by people you love. It means reading books that make you uncomfortable. It means letting go of that know-it-all pride and becoming a student again.

But freedom is on the other side of that work.

Do the Work

Reflect with honesty:

> ➤ What belief am I holding that no longer serves my growth?
> ➤ What do I spend more time doing—learning, complaining, or distracting myself?
> ➤ When was the last time I studied something that challenged me deeply?
> ➤ Who do I talk to that helps me grow intellectually?

This isn't just about gaining knowledge. It's about owning your mindset and refusing to let your thoughts run your life without your permission.

You don't need another degree. You need mental clarity. You need intellectual ownership. You need to know what you know—and unlearn what's been holding you hostage.

So before we go fix your money, your circle, your habits, or your emotions... start here.

" Upgrade your thoughts "

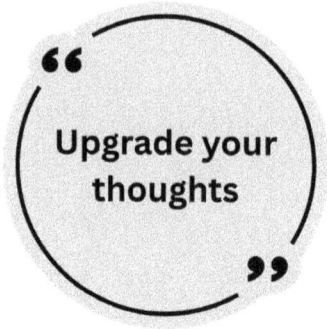

Strengthen your mind. Upgrade your thoughts. Coach your damn self—and give your future self the gift of mental freedom.

CHAPTER 3: EMOTIONAL – THE TRUTH ABOUT YOUR FEELINGS

You've been taught to "toughen up," "get over it," or "keep it moving." But here's the truth: suppressing your emotions doesn't make you stronger—it makes you stuck.

> **Your emotions aren't enemies.**

Your emotions aren't enemies. They're messengers in the emotional dimension of your life. It's not about being overly sensitive or unshakably stoic. It's about being honest. Honest about how you feel, why you feel that way, and what those feelings are trying to tell you.

This chapter is about learning to feel without falling apart—about managing your emotions without letting them manage you.

WHAT DOES "EMOTIONAL" REALLY MEAN?

It's not just about crying or staying calm under pressure. Emotional intelligence is about recognizing, understanding, and handling your feelings—especially when life gets messy. It's about being aware of what's happening inside of you so you don't explode, shut down, or sabotage the good things trying to come into your life.

It's:

➢ How you handle disappointment, anger, fear, or rejection
➢ Whether you react or respond when you're triggered
➢ Your ability to communicate your needs without shame
➢ How well you love, forgive, and let go

This is the side of you that most people don't see—but it's the one that shapes everything.

EMOTIONAL BAGGAGE VS. EMOTIONAL AWARENESS

Most of us are carrying bags we never packed. Generational trauma. Childhood wounds. Relationship residue. And we walk through life trying to smile while dragging suitcases of pain behind us. "The legendary Erykah Badu gave us the timeless track 'Bag Lady.' Do yourself a favor—take a quick pause, look up the lyrics, let them sink in, and then come back to this book right where you left off. Trust me, it'll hit different."

> **You can't move freely with baggage. But you can heal it—if you're willing to face it.**

You can't move freely with baggage. But you can heal it—if you're willing to face it.

Ask yourself:

➢ What triggers me, and why?
➢ Am I reacting to this moment—or to something from my past?
➢ Do I suppress emotions to appear "strong"?
➢ Do I give myself space to feel—or do I distract myself with busyness?

You can't heal what you won't acknowledge. Period.

EMOTIONAL HYGIENE MATTERS

Just like your body needs showers, your heart and soul need cleansing too. If you're constantly overwhelmed, irritable, numb, or disconnected, your emotional hygiene needs work.

It starts with creating habits that help you stay in tune with yourself:

➢ Journal your thoughts so they don't bottle up
➢ Talk to someone who can listen without judgment

➤ Practice saying how you really feel—even if your voice shakes

➤ Rest when your soul is tired—not just your body

➤ Clean emotions = clearer decisions. Don't let emotional clutter sabotage your peace.

STOP EMOTIONAL OUTSOURCING

You ever look to someone else to make you feel whole, worthy, or validated? That's emotional outsourcing. And it's dangerous.

No one else is responsible for your healing. Your peace. Your joy.

You are.

That doesn't mean you never lean on people—but it does mean you stop giving them the keys to your emotional well-being.

Check yourself:

➤ Do I need others to agree with me to feel secure?

> ➤ Do I blame others for how I feel?
> ➤ Do I expect someone to fix what I haven't dealt with?

Take the reins back. Your emotions are your job.

STRENGTH IS EMOTIONAL AGILITY

Let me say this clearly: strength is not emotional suppression. Strength is emotional regulation.

> " **strength is not emotional suppression. Strength is emotional regulation** "

It's knowing how to stay grounded when your world feels chaotic. It's being able to breathe through anger, cry without shame, apologize without ego, and speak truth with compassion.

Strong people feel. They just don't let feelings rule them.

Want to evolve emotionally? Start here:

> ➤ Do I pause before reacting—or lash out and regret it later?
> ➤ Can I name my emotions without judgment?
> ➤ Do I allow others to express themselves—or only want to be heard?

If you're not growing emotionally, you'll keep repeating the same cycles with different faces.

REAL TALK: UNFELT FEELINGS DON'T DIE— THEY LEAK

You think you've buried that grief, that rage, that rejection? Nah. You've just tucked it away in your body, your habits, your relationships.

Unprocessed emotions find their way out—through sarcasm, withdrawal, addiction, control, perfectionism.

Let this hit:

That thing you won't deal with is still dealing with you.

> **That thing you won't deal with is still dealing with you.**

But there's good news—you don't need to fix everything overnight. You just need to feel. To be present with your emotions without shame. To let the tears come. To let the healing begin.

Do the Work

Check in with yourself:

- ➢ What emotion have I been avoiding?
- ➢ What unhealthy coping mechanisms do I run to?

➢ Who do I need to forgive—including myself?
➢ Do I feel safe being vulnerable with anyone?

This isn't about becoming emotional. It's about becoming emotionally honest. Owning your feelings doesn't make you weak—it makes you wise.

So before we talk about building new habits, deep relationships, or powerful leadership—check your heart. Clean your emotional house. Learn to sit with your feelings without running from them.

Emotional maturity is the foundation for a fulfilled life.

Feel it. Face it. Free yourself.

CHAPTER 4: SOCIAL – THE ENERGY OF YOUR CONNECTIONS

Let's get something straight real quick: Your life isn't just built by what you do—it's shaped by who you do it with.

You weren't meant to walk this journey alone. But you also weren't meant to carry people who keep slowing you down.

The Social dimension of your life is about your relationships—your family, friends, work crew, tribe, community, all of it. It's about how you connect, communicate, give, and receive. It's the vibe, the energy, the rhythm of your circles. And if your social energy is toxic, messy, or draining... don't be surprised if your growth feels stunted.

Let's talk about the company you keep—and the version of you that shows up in those rooms.

WHAT DOES "SOCIAL" REALLY MEAN?

It's not about being popular. Or having 5,000 followers and nobody who checks on you. Social health is relational health. It's:

➢ Who pours into you—and who only pulls from you
➢ How you show up in community
➢ Whether your relationships feel safe, real, and mutual

Whether you know the difference between support and attachment

You could be the most talented person in the room—but if your circle is filled with competition, chaos, or codependency, your potential stays capped.

> 66 **if your circle is filled with competition, chaos, or codependency, your potential stays capped.** 99

THE PEOPLE IN YOUR LIFE ARE MIRRORS

Who you surround yourself with reflects how you feel about yourself. Read that again.

If you're constantly around people who:

> ➤ Drain you
> ➤ Dismiss your dreams
> ➤ Trigger your trauma
> ➤ Or always need saving

...then deep down, you might still believe that's what you deserve.

Ask yourself:

> ➤ Who in my life energizes me—and who exhausts me?
> ➤ Do I have people I can be fully myself with?
> ➤ Am I trying to be liked—or truly known?
> ➤ Do I keep relationships that feel familiar—or that feel healthy?

Your social circle should sharpen you, not shrink you.

CONNECTION OVER CLOUT

We live in a time where "networking" gets mistaken for "collecting people." But real social health isn't about stacking contacts—it's about building connections.

> 66
>
> ## We live in a time where "networking" gets mistaken for "collecting people."
>
> 99

There's a big difference between:

- ➢ Being in the room vs. belonging in the room
- ➢ Being talked to vs. being seen
- ➢ Being tolerated vs. being celebrated

Let this chapter be a wake-up call: Stop chasing crowds that don't even know you. Start building community with people who value you.

BOUNDARIES ARE LOVE, NOT REJECTION

Let's kill this myth: Setting boundaries doesn't make you mean. It makes you mature.

If you're constantly saying "yes" to keep the peace, but you're at war with yourself—you're not being nice. You're being neglectful of your own needs.

Here's how you start protecting your peace:

- ➢ Learn to say "no" without a full explanation
- ➢ Stop explaining your growth to people committed to misunderstanding you
- ➢ Prioritize mutual relationships—reciprocity isn't a luxury, it's a requirement

You don't owe unlimited access to people just because you love them. Boundaries are how love lasts.

REAL TALK: CHECK THE VIBE YOU BRING TOO

This isn't just about who you're connected to—it's about what kind of connection you are.

Ask yourself:

- ➢ Am I a safe place for others—or a source of drama?
- ➢ Do I listen to understand—or wait to reply?
- ➢ Do I uplift others—or compete with them?
- ➢ Do I gossip, ghost, or grow?

Your social dimension can't thrive if you're the one poisoning the water. Own your part. Heal your tendencies. Choose to be the kind of friend, partner, or leader you wish you had.

YOUR SOCIAL CIRCLE IS YOUR SOIL

You don't grow in isolation—but you don't grow in just any environment either.

Some people water you. Others drain you. And if you're not intentional, you'll plant your dreams in soil that was never meant to sustain them.

Here's the truth:

Not everyone is meant to go with you to your next level. And that's okay. Some people were chapters, not lifetime contracts. Appreciate the lesson. Release the weight.

> " Not everyone is meant to go with you to your next level. "

Do the Work

- ➢ Social wellness takes courage. Start with this:
- ➢ Who in my life challenges me to be better?

➢ Who have I outgrown, but haven't let go?
➢ Where am I settling for connection that costs me my peace?
➢ Am I being the kind of person I'm hoping to find?

Don't just audit your circle—upgrade your role in it.

This chapter isn't about cutting everyone off. It's about being clear about what kind of energy you want around your life, your purpose, your peace.

You deserve relationships that reflect the love, growth, and power you're cultivating. So build your tribe. Protect your peace. And remember:

➢ Your **network** is not just your **net worth**. It's your *lifeline*.
➢ Choose wisely. Love deeply. Connect intentionally.
➢ Your future is watching who you let sit at your table.

CHAPTER 5: ECONOMICAL – THE TRUTH ABOUT YOUR MONEY MINDSET

Money isn't everything—but let's not pretend it's nothing either.

You've probably heard, "Money doesn't buy happiness." Sure. But let's be real: it pays for peace, options, and the kind of freedom that stress can't survive in. And *if your financial life is out of order, it's going to ripple into every other dimension of your existence.*

> **"**
>
> **if your financial life is out of order, it's going to ripple into every other dimension of your existence.**

The Economical dimension is not just about how much money you make. It's about how you manage it, value it, and relate to it. Your money mindset is just as powerful as your income—and if you don't fix it, your bag will always come with a leak.

WHAT DOES "ECONOMICAL" REALLY MEAN?

It's not just about being frugal or having a savings account. It's:

➢ Your relationship with money—do you control it, or does it control you?
➢ How you handle resources—not just cash, but time, energy, and skills
➢ Whether you operate out of abundance or lack

How you use money: as a tool, a crutch, a mask—or a mission

This isn't about being rich. It's about being wise. Because no matter how much money you make, if your mindset stays broke, so will your life.

YOU CAN'T HEAL IN THE SAME MONEY PATTERNS THAT HURT YOU

Let's be honest: most of us were never taught how to handle money—we were just handed money and told not to waste it. But here's the thing: if you were raised in lack, chaos, or survival mode, you're probably still carrying that energy every time you get paid.

Are you:

➢ Spending to impress instead of investing to grow?
➢ Always broke the day after payday?
➢ Feeling guilty when you finally do something nice for yourself?
➢ Afraid to look at your bank account?

Your money habits are often your emotional wounds dressed up in receipts. And until you change the story you believe about money, the outcome won't change either.

SCARCITY THINKING KEEPS YOU STUCK

Scarcity is the mindset that says:

> **Scarcity thinking creates a scarcity life.**

- ➢ "There's never enough."
- ➢ "If I give, I'll lose."
- ➢ "I can't afford to invest in myself."
- ➢ "Money is hard to come by, so I better hoard it or hustle 24/7."

But here's the truth: ***Scarcity thinking creates a scarcity life.*** When you operate from fear, every financial decision becomes a trap. And fear-based money never builds freedom—it just builds more fear.

Flip the script:

➤ Start budgeting as an act of power, not punishment
➤ Save because you're building legacy, not because you're scared
➤ Invest in what multiplies, not what distracts

Abundance isn't just a number—it's a mindset.

REAL TALK: YOU DON'T HAVE A MONEY PROBLEM—YOU HAVE A DISCIPLINE PROBLEM

Listen, it's not always about how much you make. It's about what you do with what you have.

Making six figures won't help if you spend like you're proving something to people who don't even like you. And if every blessing turns into a burden because you can't manage it—you'll stay stuck in the same cycle, just with nicer stuff.

Let this sink in:

Financial peace is not a dream—it's a decision

> **Financial peace is not a dream—it's a decision**

➢ If you don't tell your money where to go, it'll disappear and leave you confused

➢ Discipline is how you keep wealth, not just how you create it

➢ Don't let lifestyle creep kill your goals. Elevation requires structure.

➢ Money Is a Tool—Not Your Identity

Some of y'all are using money to buy personality. To cover insecurities. To validate worth.

But here's the truth: If you're broke in confidence, no amount of cash can fix it. If you're rich in integrity, you're already wealthy.

Money is meant to:

➢ Build things
➢ Bless people
➢ Buy back time
➢ Fund your freedom

Not impress strangers or mask pain. Get clear on what you're using it for—and make it serve you, not the other way around.

Do the Work

It's time to check your financial pulse:

- ➤ What beliefs about money did I inherit—and are they helping or hurting?
- ➤ Do I have a clear plan for how I earn, spend, save, and give?
- ➤ Am I building legacy—or just living for the moment?
- ➤ What's one money habit I can upgrade this week?

This isn't about perfection. It's about responsibility. Because you can't talk about freedom and ignore your finances.

Own your money story. Rewrite the script. Be the first in your family to break cycles and build wealth on purpose.

You don't need to be a millionaire tomorrow. But you do need to stop living paycheck to panic.

Money is not the enemy. Mismanagement is.

So fix the leaks. Watch your words. Upgrade your habits.

And remember: You're not just building income—you're building impact.

Make it count.

CHAPTER 6: SPIRITUAL – THE POWER BENEATH THE SURFACE

Let's get this out the way early: Spirituality is not religion.

You can go to church every Sunday and still feel lost. You can quote scripture and still lack peace. This chapter? It's not about rules—it's about roots.

The Spiritual dimension of your life is your core— your why, your inner compass, your connection to something greater than yourself. It's not about what you say with your mouth—it's about what anchors your soul when everything else falls apart.

Because when life hits hard (and it will), money won't save you. Friends may not show up. But your spirit? That's what keeps you standing.

WHAT DOES "SPIRITUAL" REALLY MEAN?

Spiritual doesn't mean mystical. It doesn't mean spooky. And it sure doesn't mean perfect.

It means:

➢ You're connected to your Creator, your purpose, and your inner peace
➢ You're grounded, even when life is chaotic
➢ You live by principles, not pressure
➢ You've got something inside you that doesn't break when the world around you does

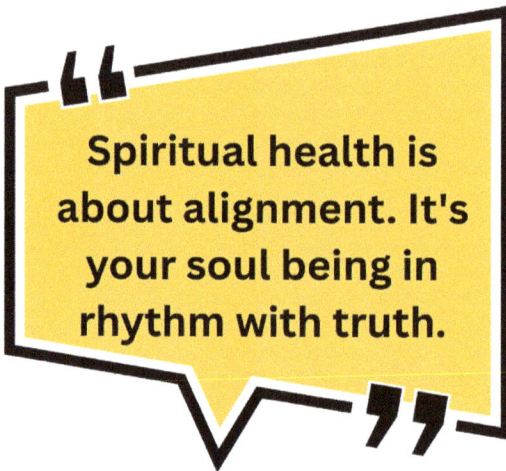

> **Spiritual health is about alignment. It's your soul being in rhythm with truth.**

Spiritual health is about alignment. It's your soul being in rhythm with truth. It's quiet strength, sacred rest, and divine direction.

YOU'RE NOT JUST FLESH AND HUSTLE

This world will have you thinking your worth is based on your productivity, your grind, your likes, your status. But deep down, you know: there's more to you than what people see.

You're not just a body. You're not just a brand. You're not just a provider, a parent, a partner.

You're a spirit wrapped in skin—and your soul needs care too.

Ask yourself:

➤ When was the last time I felt spiritually full—not just busy or distracted?
➤ Do I make space for stillness, reflection, prayer, or meditation?
➤ Am I living by purpose—or just surviving through routine?
➤ Do I trust that I'm being guided—or do I think I have to carry everything alone?

If you don't feed your spirit, your life will starve—even if it looks full.

YOU CAN'T HUSTLE YOUR WAY INTO WHOLENESS

Let's kill the myth: More work won't fix a weary soul.

You could have the perfect business plan, flawless branding, and multiple streams of income—but still be hollow inside. Why? ***Because spiritual hunger can't be filled with physical success.***

> **Because spiritual hunger can't be filled with physical success.**

Some of y'all are running on fumes. And it's not because you're lazy—it's because your soul needs rest, not more hustle.

Here's your permission:

- ➢ Rest is holy
- ➢ Boundaries are sacred
- ➢ Stillness is strategy

➢ Silence is medicine
➢ Don't just chase the dream. Consult the Source.

REAL TALK: DON'T JUST PRAY FOR A BLESSING—BE IN POSITION TO RECEIVE ONE

We love to say, "I'm waiting on God." But let's be honest—sometimes God's been waiting on you to get aligned. To release what no longer serves you. To surrender control. To trust deeper. To listen when it's quiet.

Spiritual maturity means you don't just ask for things—you prepare for them. It means:

➢ You trust divine timing, not your ego's deadlines
➢ You seek wisdom, not just wins
➢ You move with integrity, even when nobody's watching
➢ You're led by peace, not pressure

Faith without action is fantasy. Action without faith is anxiety.

You need both.

PROTECT YOUR SPIRIT LIKE YOU PROTECT YOUR PASSWORDS

You wouldn't give everyone access to your bank account. So why let just anybody speak into your life?

Spiritual boundaries matter. Not every voice is from God. Not every vibe is safe. Not every opportunity is divine. Be discerning.

Check your inputs:

- ➤ What are you watching, listening to, absorbing?
- ➤ Who are you trusting with your peace?
- ➤ Are your spiritual habits feeding your growth—or numbing your guilt?

Your spirit deserves sacred space. Guard it like your future depends on it—because it does.

Do the Work

This isn't about becoming "more spiritual" so you can impress people. It's about getting real with yourself and returning to your center.

Start here:

- ➢ What spiritual practices bring me peace and clarity?
- ➢ When do I feel most connected to God, Source, or the divine?
- ➢ What am I clinging to that I need to surrender?
- ➢ Do I live in alignment with my values—or just say I do?

Spiritual wellness isn't about being perfect. It's about being present.

It's about listening deeper. Loving fuller. Living lighter.

It's remembering that your power doesn't come from what you have—but from who you are.

So breathe. Pray. Meditate. Journal. Worship. Reflect.

Whatever your practice—make it personal, make it intentional, make it consistent.

You are more than muscle, mind, or money. You are spirit.

And when your spirit is strong, you become unstoppable.

CHAPTER 7: KNOW WHERE YOU STAND

Before you can build the life you want, you need to face where you really are.

No filters. No sugarcoating. No more lying to yourself just to feel better in the moment.

You've done the work. You've read the chapters. You've set the goals. But now? It's time to take inventory—with brutal honesty.

Because you can't grow from where you wish you were. You can only grow from where you actually are.

THIS IS YOUR REALITY CHECK

Here's the deal:

You're going to rate yourself from **0 to 10** in each of the six dimensions—Physical, Intellectual, Emotional, Social, Economical, and Spiritual. Not based on perfection. Not based on where you used to be. But based on how close you are to the person you truly want to become.

Then, you'll write a short explanation—just a sentence or two—to own your truth.

After that, you'll total the scores, divide by 60, and multiply by 100 to get a percentage.

This number?

That's how much of your full potential you're currently living.

Not to shame you. To show you. Because you can't hit a target you haven't identified.

Let's get into it.

PHYSICAL (0–10)

How close are you to your ideal level of energy, health, strength, and physical care?

My score: _____

Why I gave myself this score:

_____

_____

_____

INTELLECTUAL (0–10)

How close are you to the level of mental sharpness, learning, growth, and clarity you want?

My score: _____

Why I gave myself this score:

_____

_____

_____

EMOTIONAL (0–10)

How close are you to mastering your emotions, expressing yourself honestly, and feeling emotionally balanced?

My score: _____

Why I gave myself this score:

_____

_____

_____

SOCIAL (0–10)

How close are you to having healthy, supportive, meaningful relationships with people who challenge and uplift you?

My score: _____

Why I gave myself this score:

_____

_____

_____

ECONOMICAL (0–10)

How close are you to feeling in control of your money, building wealth, and making financial decisions that align with your goals?

My score: _____

Why I gave myself this score:

_____

_____

_____

SPIRITUAL (0–10)

How close are you to feeling grounded in your faith, purpose, inner peace, and connection to something greater than yourself?

My score: _____

Why I gave myself this score:

_____

_____

_____

Now Add It Up

Add all six scores together:

Total: _____ / 60

Then divide your total by 60, and multiply by 100 to get your percentage.

I am currently operating at _____% of the person I truly want to be.

This Is Your Starting Point

This number is not who you'll always be. It's just where you are right now.

Maybe you're at 73%. Maybe 42%. Maybe 88%.

Whatever it is—own it. Don't flinch. Don't fake it. And definitely don't beat yourself up.

This is your GPS location. And you can't get to where you're going without knowing where you're standing.

This number is your truth.

And from this moment on, you've got a baseline. A benchmark. A beginning.

Now that you've faced the real you—

You can finally go build the next you.

REAL TALK BEFORE YOU MOVE ON:

You don't have to be at 100% to make impact.

You just have to be honest, intentional, and willing to take the next step.

The goal is not perfection. The goal is progress with purpose.

Now that you know where you stand, the question is:

What are you going to do about it?

Let's get it, Coach. You're no longer reacting. You're rebuilding.

Your starting point is set. Let's go.

CHAPTER 8: S.W.O.T. – CONFRONTING THE TRUTH WITH COURAGE

Let's keep it all the way real: You can't fix what you won't face.

You've explored your Physical, Intellectual, Emotional, Social, Economical, and Spiritual dimensions—but now it's time to take inventory.

This chapter isn't about judgment. It's about clarity.

Because clarity creates power. And power creates movement.

S.W.O.T. stands for Strengths, Weaknesses, Opportunities, and Threats. And if you're serious about becoming who you were designed to be, you need to know where you stand—so you can take command.

S – STRENGTHS

What are you doing well? Where are you consistent? Where are you most powerful and most grounded?

Let's dig in:

Physical

What's one healthy habit I've maintained consistently?

_____

_____

_____

Where does my body feel strong and energized?

_____

_____

_____

What physical ability am I grateful to still have?

_____

_____

_____

Intellectual

What topics light my brain up?

_____

_____

_____

Where am I a fast learner?

_____

_____

_____

What's a decision I made recently that I'm proud of?

_____

_____

_____

Emotional

How have I grown emotionally over the past year?

_____

_____

_____

What's one emotion I've learned to manage better?

_____

_____

_____

Who or what brings me peace?

_____

_____

_____

Social

Who in my life truly supports and uplifts me?

_____

_____

_____

Where do I feel the most seen and valued?

_____

_____

_____

What's one way I contribute positively to others?

_____

_____

Economical

What financial habits are helping me grow?

_____

_____

_____

What have I done well with money this year?

_____

_____

_____

What resource do I manage wisely?

_____

_____

_____

Spiritual

When do I feel most connected to God or Source?

_____

_____

_____

What spiritual practice has kept me grounded?

_____

_____

_____

Where in my life do I feel led, not just lucky?

_____

_____

_____

W – WEAKNESSES

Let's be honest. This is where most people want to skip ahead—but you won't heal what you hide.

Physical

Where am I ignoring my health or pushing my limits?

_____

_____

_____

What habits are draining my energy instead of restoring it?

_____

_____

_____

What have I avoided dealing with physically?

_____

_____

_____

_____

Intellectual

Where am I mentally lazy or stuck in autopilot?

_____

_____

_____

What belief or idea is keeping me small?

_____

_____

_____

Am I afraid to admit when I don't know something?

_____

_____

_____

Emotional

What triggers me consistently—and why?

_____

_____

_____

Where do I still shut down, lash out, or bottle up?

_____

_____

_____

Who haven't I forgiven—especially myself?

_____

_____

_____

Social

Who do I keep around out of fear, not growth?

_____

_____

_____

Am I afraid of being alone, so I settle for less?

_____

_____

_____

How do I show up in relationships when I'm hurting?

_____

_____

_____

Economical

Where is my money going that doesn't align with my goals?

_____

_____

_____

What do I avoid financially out of fear or shame?

_____

_____

_____

Am I making emotional purchases instead of intentional investments?

_____

_____

_____

Spiritual

When do I feel disconnected from my purpose?

_____

_____

_____

What spiritual truths have I ignored?

_____

_____

_____

Do I treat God like a backup plan or my foundation?

_____

_____

_____

O – OPPORTUNITIES

Growth lives here. This is the space where alignment, awareness, and faith collide.

Physical

What's one small upgrade I could make to my health today?

_____

_____

_____

What does my body need that I've been too busy to give it?

_____

_____

_____

How can I increase my energy naturally?

_____

_____

_____

_____

Intellectual

What skill or subject should I finally learn?

_____

_____

_____

What book, course, or podcast could challenge my thinking?

_____

_____

_____

Who could mentor me mentally or professionally?

_____

_____

_____

Emotional

What new way of expressing myself could free me emotionally?

_____

_____

_____

What practice could help me regulate my emotions better?

_____

_____

_____

Who deserves a heartfelt conversation?

_____

_____

_____

Social

Who should I be spending more time with?

_____

_____

_____

What community could I plug into that nurtures my growth?

_____

_____

_____

What boundary could help me feel more whole?

_____

_____

_____

Economical

What income stream could I start, grow, or scale?

_____
_____
_____

Where can I start saving, investing, or giving intentionally?

_____
_____
_____

Who can I learn from financially?

_____
_____
_____

Spiritual

What would deepen my spiritual walk?

_____

_____

_____

What spiritual community, practice, or truth do I need to explore?

_____

_____

_____

Where is God inviting me to trust more?

_____

_____

_____

T – THREATS

This is where you call out the stuff that can sabotage your progress if you don't stay alert. Think: distractions, bad habits, patterns, people, fear, ego.

Physical

What physical patterns are slowly harming me?

_____

_____

_____

Where am I ignoring warning signs?

_____

_____

_____

What could become a health crisis if I don't address it now?

_____

_____

_____

_____

Intellectual

What content am I consuming that dulls my thinking?

_____

_____

_____

Who do I listen to that feeds fear or ignorance?

_____

_____

_____

Where am I overthinking and under-executing?

_____

_____

_____

Emotional

What emotion has the power to throw me completely off track?

_____

_____

_____

What wound keeps showing up in my decisions?

_____

_____

_____

Who has access to me that shouldn't?

_____

_____

_____

Social

What relationships are draining or distracting me?

_____

_____

_____

Where do I still people-please to my own detriment?

_____

_____

_____

Who am I trying to save instead of letting go?

_____

_____

_____

Economical

What habits or mindsets are keeping me in lack?

_____

_____

_____

What am I doing with money that I wouldn't want anyone to see?

_____

_____

_____

Where am I vulnerable financially?

_____

_____

_____

Spiritual

What causes me to drift spiritually?

_____

_____

_____

What voices are louder than God's in my life?

_____

_____

_____

Where am I trying to control instead of surrendering?

_____

_____

_____

FINAL THOUGHT: AWARENESS IS THE FIRST KEY TO FREEDOM

This chapter isn't about perfection. It's about precision.

You can't grow what you won't measure. You can't heal what you won't name.

So take your time. Sit with the questions. Be honest, not heroic.

Because the more truth you're willing to face—

The more power you're ready to activate.

Let's get to work, and let's get free.

CHAPTER 9: D.A.B.D.A. – GRIEVING THE OLD YOU

Let's get into something nobody really tells you:

Becoming your best self comes with grief.

Not because you lost—but because you let go.

When you start changing your life, you don't just leave behind bad habits.

 You leave behind comfort. Identity. People. Old versions of yourself.

And even if you know it's for the best, there's still a part of you that's going to mourn it.

This chapter is about what that mourning looks like—and how to get through it without quitting.

 You're not just building a better future. You're laying to rest a former version of you. And that process is real.

Welcome to **D.A.B.D.A**. — the 5 emotional stages of grief:

DENIAL – "THIS CAN'T BE HAPPENING"

When you first commit to real change—breaking a cycle, ending a toxic relationship, quitting that job, showing up for yourself consistently—you may resist the very thing you asked for.

You'll hear yourself say:

- ➤ "Maybe it wasn't that bad."
- ➤ "Maybe I'm overthinking this."
- ➤ "I can't really start over... can I?"

This is your comfort zone begging for another chance.

But don't fall for it. Denial is just fear dressed up as logic.

Ask yourself:

- ➤ Am I rejecting the new because it's unfamiliar?
- ➤ What truth am I pretending not to see?
- ➤ What part of me is afraid to move forward?

Denial doesn't protect you—it delays you.

ANGER – "WHY DOES THIS HURT SO MUCH?"

Change comes with growing pains. And anger is usually the first loud emotion that shows up.

You might feel mad that:

➢ People didn't support you.
➢ You stayed in the wrong situation too long.
➢ You're struggling with something others seem to do easily.

This isn't weakness—it's release.

 Anger is your soul clearing space. Don't let it poison you, but don't ignore it either.

Ask yourself:

➢ Who or what am I really mad at?
➢ Am I blaming others instead of facing my own decisions?
➢ What's underneath the anger—hurt, disappointment, betrayal?

Feel it. Process it. But don't live in it.

BARGAINING – "CAN I JUST GO BACK FOR A SECOND?"

This is the trap of almost-letting-go.

You start negotiating with your old life:

➢ "Maybe I can do both."
➢ "What if I just change a little?"
➢ "Let me talk to them one more time."

Bargaining is your ego trying to keep one foot in the past.

It's your way of softening the loss—but all it really does is delay your progress.

Ask yourself:

➢ What am I afraid of losing completely?
➢ Am I holding onto crumbs because I'm scared of the feast?
➢ What deal am I trying to make with a version of me that no longer exists?

You can't walk into your new life dragging old habits behind you. Let them go.

DEPRESSION – "WHY DOES THIS FEEL SO HEAVY?"

This is the quiet part. The part where the reality of change sinks in. The hype is gone. The decision is made. But the grief? It lingers.

You'll feel:

➢ Lonely even if you're not alone.
➢ Disconnected from people who used to feel close.
➢ Sad, tired, or even numb.

This is the death of identity. And that's no small thing.

But here's the truth: It's okay to grieve your old life.

It doesn't mean you want it back—it means you're honoring what used to be.

Ask yourself:

➢ What am I really mourning?
➢ What needs to be healed, not hidden?
➢ Who can I talk to about this without shame?

This phase is temporary. Let yourself feel—so you can move forward freely.

ACCEPTANCE – "I'M STILL HERE. AND I'M READY."

This is where the light starts breaking through.

You stop clinging to who you were—and start becoming who you are.

You'll feel:

- ➤ More clear, even if still a little scared.
- ➤ More stable, even if everything's not perfect.
- ➤ More whole, because you're no longer fragmented by pretending.

Acceptance doesn't mean you like what happened.

 It means you've decided to live, grow, and build anyway.

Ask yourself:

If you're truly transforming, there will be moments where it feels like something died.

That's because it did: your excuses, your coping mechanisms, your attachments, your "almosts."

So if it feels heavy—it's not because you're weak.

It's because you're shedding a version of you that can't survive in your next level.

Let it go with love. Mourn if you need to.

But don't turn back.

Do the Work

Reflect honestly:

- ➤ What part of me am I grieving right now?
- ➤ What stage am I currently sitting in—Denial, Anger, Bargaining, Depression, or Acceptance?
- ➤ What support do I need in this process?

➢ How can I honor my growth while letting go of my past?

This chapter isn't just about emotions. It's about evolution.

It's about recognizing that transformation costs something—and being willing to pay the price.

Grieve it. Grow from it.

Because on the other side of loss is liberation.

You're not just changing.

You're resurrecting.

CHAPTER 10: S.M.A.R.T. – GOALS THAT ACTUALLY GET YOU SOMEWHERE

Let's be honest: most people don't fail because they don't want change.

They fail because their goals are vague, impulsive, or straight-up unrealistic.

Saying "I want to be better" sounds noble—but it's not a strategy.

If you want real results, you need real structure. And that's where S.M.A.R.T. goals come in.

This chapter is about turning your intentions into action.

 No more wishful thinking. No more floating through life.

We're setting goals that actually move the needle in your Physical, Intellectual, Emotional, Social, Economical, and Spiritual dimensions.

WHAT MAKES A GOAL S.M.A.R.T.?

Before you write down anything, let's break down the framework:

- ➢ **S – Specific:** What exactly do you want to achieve? No fluff.
- ➢ **M – Measurable:** How will you know when it's done?
- ➢ **A – Achievable:** Is it realistic given your current time, energy, and resources?
- ➢ **R – Relevant:** Does it align with the life you're building?
- ➢ **T – Time-Bound:** When's the deadline? Put a date on it.

If your goal doesn't pass the S.M.A.R.T. test, it's just a hope dressed up as a plan.

TIME TO SET 3 GOALS IN EACH AREA OF YOUR LIFE

Don't rush this. Go deep. Think beyond what's trending. Think about what your future self is begging you to commit to today.

1. Physical – Your Body Is the Foundation

Your health is your first wealth. Period. Set goals that honor your strength, energy, and longevity.

Write 3 SMART goals:

_____

_____

_____

Examples:

- ➢ Drink 64 oz of water every day for the next 30 days
- ➢ Walk 3 times a week for 45 minutes
- ➢ Schedule and complete an annual physical exam by [insert date]

2. Intellectual – Sharpen the Weapon

Your mind is your greatest tool. Don't let it get dull. Stretch it, challenge it, evolve it.

Write 3 SMART goals:

_____

_____

_____

Examples:

- ➢ Read one non-fiction book a month for 6 months
- ➢ Complete a course on [topic] by [insert date]
- ➢ Replace 30 minutes of social media with a podcast or article 5 days a week

3. Emotional – Master the Inside Game

Your peace is priceless. Let's build emotional intelligence, resilience, and healing on purpose.

Write 3 SMART goals:

_____

_____

_____

Examples:

- ➤ Start therapy and commit to 6 weekly sessions
- ➤ Journal every morning for 10 minutes for the next 21 days
- ➤ Identify and name emotions daily before reacting

4. Social – Build the Right Circle

You're not meant to do life alone—but you are meant to be selective. Let's upgrade your connections.

Write 3 SMART goals:

_____

_____

_____

Examples:

- ➢ Call or meet with one uplifting friend every week
- ➢ Join a new group, class, or community this month
- ➢ Set a boundary with someone who drains you by [insert date]

5. Economical – Get in Financial Position

No more being confused or careless with your coins. It's time to manage your money with purpose.

Write 3 SMART goals:

_____

_____

_____

Examples:

- ➢ Save $500 in an emergency fund within 3 months
- ➢ Pay off [specific debt] by [insert date]
- ➢ Track every expense for 30 days using a budgeting app

6. Spiritual – Stay Anchored, Not Just Ambitious

Success means nothing if your soul is starving. Let's build from the inside out.

Write 3 SMART goals:

_____

_____

_____

Examples:

- ➢ Spend 10 minutes in prayer, meditation, or devotion each morning
- ➢ Attend a spiritual gathering, church, or group biweekly

> ➤ Fast from distractions (TV, social media, etc.) one day a week for 4 weeks

REAL TALK: GOALS WITHOUT STRUCTURE BECOME STRESS

This is where most people mess up—they dream big but plan small.

You can't manifest what you won't manage.

You've got to track, adjust, and check in with your goals regularly. Otherwise, they fade into the background noise of life.

Your goals aren't just tasks. They're agreements with your future self.

So write them. Review them. And hold yourself accountable like your destiny depends on it— because it does.

Do the Work

✓ Have you written 3 clear S.M.A.R.T. goals in each dimension?

✓ Are your goals connected to the person you're becoming—not just the person you've been?

✓ Do your goals stretch you without breaking you?

If yes, you're on the right path.

 If no—pause, go back, and get real.

This isn't a game. It's your life.

And your goals? They're the bricks in the road that leads to everything you want.

CHAPTER 11: T.A.H.C.D. – WHY YOUR LIFE MOVES THE WAY IT DOES

Let me put it to you plain:

You don't just end up somewhere. You build the road to it. Thought by thought. Step by step.

Most people blame life for what their mind produced. But your outcomes didn't appear out of thin air—they followed a system, whether you knew it or not. And if you want to change where you're headed, you've got to change what you're feeding.

That's where **T.A.H.C.D.** comes in:

Thought → Action → Habit → Character → Destiny

You want a better life? Don't just pray for it.

Trace it. Track it. Train for it.

T – THOUGHT: EVERY OUTCOME STARTS IN THE MIND

What you think determines what you do—even if you're not aware of it.

Thoughts are seeds. And guess what? Your life is the harvest.

You can't grow peace from seeds of chaos. You can't expect greatness while replaying garbage.

Ask yourself:

- ➢ What's my dominant thought pattern each day—hope or fear?
- ➢ Do I think with discipline, or let my mind run wild?
- ➢ Are my thoughts helping me build—or making me self-destruct?

Shift your mindset. Shift your momentum.

A – ACTION: THINKING AIN'T ENOUGH

You can journal, vision board, and manifest all day—but if you don't act, nothing changes.

Your thoughts inform your next move. But action turns thought into proof.

Ask yourself:

- ➢ What action am I avoiding because of fear or laziness?
- ➢ What's one small step I could take today that aligns with my purpose?
- ➢ Do I move with intention—or emotion?

Consistency beats intensity. Don't wait for the perfect day. Do something now.

H – HABIT: WHAT YOU REPEAT, YOU BECOME

You don't rise to the level of your potential—you fall to the level of your systems.

And your habits? That's your system on display.

Your life is a collection of small, repeated actions. The things you do without thinking are the things that are building your future—or breaking it.

Ask yourself:

> ➤ What do I do every day that's silently shaping me?
> ➤ What habit is keeping me stuck?
> ➤ What habit could unlock the next level for me?

Your results are not random—they're repeated.

C – CHARACTER: THE REAL YOU SHOWS UP HERE

Character isn't what people see—it's who you are when no one's looking.

It's your integrity, your values, your non-negotiables. And make no mistake: your habits are shaping your character in real time.

Ask yourself:

> ➤ Do I keep my word to others—but break promises to myself?
> ➤ Can I be trusted when there's nothing to gain?
> ➤ Does my life reflect what I say I believe?

Character is your spiritual credit score. Protect it.

D – DESTINY: YOU'RE NOT LUCKY, YOU'RE ALIGNED

You don't stumble into destiny.

You walk into it—or you miss it—based on everything before it.

Your thoughts → shaped your actions → built your habits → formed your character… and that's what delivered you to your current reality.

Ask yourself:

> ➤ Is my current life a reflection of who I want to be—or who I settled for being?

> ➤ What kind of future am I building with my daily choices?
> ➤ Am I reacting to life—or creating it?

You are not a victim of circumstance—you're a co-creator of your future.

REAL TALK: YOUR LIFE HAS A BLUEPRINT—AND YOU WROTE IT

Whether you realize it or not, you've already followed this path.

Maybe with chaos. Maybe with clarity. But the pattern was there.

The question is: Are you going to keep building blindly... or finally build intentionally?

Your **thoughts** are the **soil**.

Your **actions** are the **seeds**.

Your **habits** are the **roots**.

Your **character** is the **tree**.

And your **destiny**? That's the **fruit**.

Do the Work

This chapter isn't for skimming. Sit with it. Be real.

Answer these:

- ➤ What toxic thought has shaped too much of my life?
- ➤ What action have I been delaying that would change everything?
- ➤ What habit no longer belongs in my next season?
- ➤ What kind of person do I want to be, not just appear to be?
- ➤ What do I want my destiny to look like—and am I building toward it?

You've got the blueprint now.

You can no longer say "I don't know how."

It's time to take responsibility for the rhythm of your life.

Not just wishful thinking.

Not just momentary hype.

But intentional, layered, unapologetic transformation.

Chapter 11 is next.

And it's all about the "How"—a strategy-driven breakdown called I.D.E.A.L.S.O.L.V.E.

We're going from inner power to external execution. Let's finish strong.

CHAPTER 12: I.D.E.A.L.S.O.L.V.E. – HOW TO MAKE TRANSFORMATION STICK

You've reflected. You've reset. You've faced your truth in every dimension.

But now it's time to answer the real question: How do I actually live this out?

Because inspiration fades. Motivation runs out. But execution?

That's what creates legacy.

This chapter is your how-to blueprint. It's not a magic formula—it's a framework for momentum. When you feel stuck, overwhelmed, unsure what to do next—come back here.

Welcome to **I.D.E.A.L.S.O.L.V.E.**

Ten steps. One mission: solve what's been keeping you stuck.

I – IDENTIFY THE PROBLEM

Call it what it is. Be honest about what's really not working.

Is it a cycle? A fear? A belief? A habit?

What are you avoiding that's costing you peace?

You can't fix what you won't face. Name it—don't dance around it.

D – DEFINE THE PROBLEM CLEARLY

Get specific. Vagueness is the enemy of progress.

"I'm overwhelmed" becomes → "I don't know how to manage my schedule."

"I'm broke" becomes → "I'm spending more than I earn."

The clearer the problem, the sharper your strategy.

E – EXPLORE POSSIBLE SOLUTIONS

Brainstorm. Think big, think practical, think outside your normal routine.

What have you never tried because it felt too uncomfortable?

Who has done what you're trying to do?

Don't limit your options. Growth lives in possibility.

A – ASSESS EACH SOLUTION

Now check the weight. Which solutions are doable, sustainable, and aligned?

What resources will this take (time, money, energy)?

Will it push you forward—or just keep you busy?

Don't confuse motion with progress.

L – LAYOUT YOUR PLAN

Turn your top choice into a step-by-step plan. No more vague goals—write it out.

What's Step 1?

What will I do each day/week to stay on track?

Plans don't guarantee success—but failing to plan guarantees struggle.

S – START THE SOLUTION

Execution time. No overthinking. No waiting for perfect.

Start messy if you must—just start.

Take one action within the next 24 hours.

Movement breeds clarity. Action activates growth.

O – OBSERVE THE PROGRESS

Track what's happening. Check your results and your mindset.

Am I getting closer or just getting busy?

What's working? What's draining me?

Don't be afraid to pivot. Self-awareness is power.

L – LOCK IN WHAT WORKS

Once something is helping—anchor it. Turn it into a habit. Make it part of your lifestyle.

How can I make this a system, not just a phase?

What boundaries or routines protect this progress?

When you find what works—protect it at all costs.

V – VERIFY THE EFFECTIVENESS

Give it time, but don't keep doing something that's not producing fruit.

Has my life improved in this area?

Would the future version of me say, "Keep going"?

Proof > hype. Let results lead you, not emotion.

E – EVALUATE WHAT'S NEXT

Once you've solved one problem, don't stop.

Ask yourself: What's the next thing I need to face?

What other area of my life needs this same energy?

Where am I still shrinking when I should be showing up?

Progress isn't a destination—it's a rhythm. Keep evolving.

REAL TALK: STOP GETTING READY. STAY READY.

This framework? It's not just about healing. It's about handling life with strategy.

So the next time chaos hits—or confusion creeps in—you won't spiral. You'll solve.

You'll:

➢ Know what's wrong
➢ Name it without shame
➢ Create a strategy
➢ Take real steps
➢ Lock it in
➢ And keep it pushing

That's how you win. Quietly. Consistently. Completely.

Do the Work

Right now:

Pick one challenge you're facing.

Walk it through the I.D.E.A.L.S.O.L.V.E. framework.

Take action within 24 hours. Not next week. Now.

CHAPTER 13: FINAL WORDS: FROM SURVIVAL TO STRATEGY

You didn't just read a book—you stepped into a process that dared you to face yourself at every level. This wasn't about hype or surface-level motivation. This was a full reset—body, mind, heart, soul, and strategy. You were invited to stop surviving and start building with purpose. And now, you've got the blueprint in your hands.

It all started with P.I.E.S.E.S., the six dimensions that make up who you are: Physical, Intellectual, Emotional, Social, Economical, and Spiritual. You paused and took a hard, honest look at your life— how your body feels, how your mind works, how your emotions show up, how your relationships are serving you (or not), how you're handling your money, and how grounded you are spiritually. This holistic view gave you clarity—not just about what's broken, but about what's worth building.

Then you stepped into S.W.O.T.—a reality check. You explored your Strengths, your Weaknesses, your Opportunities for growth, and the Threats keeping you stuck. You moved from emotional fog into self-awareness, and with that came power. You stopped guessing and started owning your truth.

But you couldn't build a new life without grieving the old one. That's where D.A.B.D.A. came in. You realized that growth often feels like loss—loss of comfort, habits, people, and identity. You walked through Denial, Anger, Bargaining, Depression, and Acceptance—not just as concepts, but as emotional checkpoints in your transformation. You understood that to level up, you have to let go.

Next, you ditched vague goals and created structure with S.M.A.R.T. goals—Specific, Measurable, Achievable, Relevant, and Time-bound. You set three goals in each life dimension so that every part of you would grow in sync. You stopped saying "I want better" and started defining what "better" actually looks like—and how to get there.

You learned that your life isn't random. Chapter 10 broke it down with T.A.H.C.D.: Thought becomes Action. Action becomes Habit. Habit becomes Character. Character becomes Destiny. You realized that your outcomes aren't accidents—they're patterns. And once you saw that, you gained the power to rewrite your future, starting from your thoughts.

And finally, in Chapter 11, you got the how. I.D.E.A.L.S.O.L.V.E. became your step-by-step blueprint for solving anything that stands in your way. You now know how to Identify and Define the problem, Explore and Assess solutions, Layout a plan, Start the process, Observe your results, Lock in what works, Verify the effectiveness, and Evaluate what's next. It's not just about progress—it's about sustainable, repeatable growth.

So now what?

Now, you live this. You apply it. You make this your lifestyle. You're not surviving anymore—you're building with intention. You have the tools to coach yourself through every season, every setback, every opportunity. You don't need another pep talk. You've already done the hardest part: you faced the mirror and didn't flinch.

You've seen who you were. You've grieved what you had to let go. You've clarified your goals. You've understood the mechanics of change. And you've been given a plan that works.

So from this point forward, never let the old version of you negotiate with your future. Don't wait for perfect conditions. Don't wait for permission. Don't wait for motivation. The foundation is already in you. The path is already clear. Your future is watching.

Now go build it—on purpose, with power, and without apology.

You're no longer surviving. You're strategizing for greatness.

JOURNAL SECTION

_____

_____

_____

_____

_____

_____

_____

_____

_____

_____

_____

_____

_____

_____

AUTHOR'S BIO

Clifton Roy Jr. is a transformative business strategist, branding expert, and leadership coach known for his bold, no-excuses approach to personal and professional growth. As the founder of **PEN Business Solutions**, Clifton has helped entrepreneurs, creatives, and small business owners bring clarity to chaos by building brands that are not only visually powerful but also rooted in purpose, strategy, and sustainability.

With over two decades of experience across military service, leadership development, creative direction, and consulting, Clifton brings a rare blend of discipline, authenticity, and street-smart wisdom to every room he enters. His journey from surviving hardship to strategically navigating multiple successful ventures fuels his passion for empowering others to do the same—without fluff, and without waiting on permission.

Clifton believes that coaching isn't about hand-holding—it's about handing people the tools they need to take charge of their own lives. That philosophy is the heartbeat of his book, ***SOS – Survival Or Strategy: HOW TO COACH YOUR DAMN SELF***, where he distills his most powerful coaching principles into a self-paced guide that saves readers hundreds in coaching fees while delivering the mindset shift they truly need.

A proud veteran, creative thinker, and community advocate, Clifton has mentored countless individuals and teams, helping them recognize when they're stuck in survival mode and guiding them toward strategic action. His style is honest, his insights are actionable, and his impact is undeniable.

When he's not speaking truth into people's lives or building legacy-driven brands, Clifton can be found pouring into his family, mentoring up-and-coming entrepreneurs, or staying grounded through music, storytelling, and service. His motto is simple: *You already have what it takes—now learn how to use it.*

Whether through the pages of a book, the lens of a brand, or the fire of a coaching session, **Clifton Roy Jr. is on a mission to wake people up to their own power—and show them how to move with purpose**.

CONTACT OR FOLLOW ME

If you're seeking personal or professional coaching, dynamic speaking engagements, publishing support, or expert help with marketing, branding, or training — we'd love to connect. Reach out to us through any of the following channels:

Facebook: I'm-King Roy & PEN Business Solutions

Instagram: everyonecallsmeking & PEN Business Solutions

TikTok: everyonecallsmeking & PEN Business Solutions

Website: www.penbusinesssolutions.com

Email: info@penbusinesssolutions.com

Phone: (337) 222-3363

www.ingramcontent.com/pod-product-compliance
Lightning Source LLC
Chambersburg PA
CBHW040407110426
42812CB00011B/2484

*9 7 9 8 9 9 9 3 2 3 9 0 3 *